Got To SHINE

Got To SHINE

A GUIDEBOOK FOR TRUE HEALTH AND SUSTAINED WELLNESS IN THE 21ST CENTURY

Wally Taylor MD

ISBN: 1508838283
ISBN 13: 9781508838289
Library of Congress Control Number: 2015904417
CreateSpace Independent Publishing Platform
North Charleston, South Carolina

This guidebook is dedicated to the many patients I have seen over the years, especially those who had fallen through the cracks of the traditional Western approach to healthcare and continued to fight to regain and maintain their true health and sustained wellness.

Table of Contents

Preface

A gradual revolution is expanding in American medicine today. This revolution is largely motivated by a changing public that is demanding a more individualized, natural, and holistic approach to health care. The public is voicing with increased loudness the perception that the traditional fee-for-service, prescription-based approach to treatment has left many individuals still struggling with symptoms and disabilities that are not being adequately addressed. This guidebook is a journey through my own personal transition into this new health-care universe, and it explores some of my views on the origins of this new system. I also present to the interested reader some of the solutions to many of the difficult problems I have learned to deal with over a thirty-five-year career in medicine.

Medical Disclaimer

All the content of this book was created for informational purposes only. The purpose of this book is to promote broad consumer understanding and knowledge of various health topics. The content is not intended to be a substitute for professional medical advice, diagnosis, or treatment. Always seek the advice of your physician or other qualified health provider with any questions you may have regarding a medical condition. Never disregard professional medical advice or delay in seeking it because of something you have read in this book. If you think you may have a medical emergency, call your doctor, go to the emergency department, or call 911 immediately. The author does not recommend or endorse any specific tests, physicians, products, procedures, opinions, or other information that may be mentioned within this book. The information contained in this book is not intended nor implied to be a substitute for professional medical advice and is provided for educational purposes only. The reader assumes full responsibility for how she/he chooses to use this information. The information in this book should not be used as a substitute for the care and knowledge that your physician or other licensed care provider can provide you.

CHAPTER 1

A New Paradigm in Health Care

Western medicine is the style of medicine taught to and practiced by most physicians and many other health-care providers in the United States and Canada. Much of Western medicine today can be further categorized as the episodic model of care—one disease, one cause, one solution. This style of medicine is also sometimes referred to as disease-based, sickness-based, symptom-based, Band-Aid, or drive-through medicine. In this system, each interaction of the patient with the care provider is a single episode or a start-to-finish treatment of a single problem. This style of care lends itself best to problems of sudden and discrete causes that can be easily identified and dealt with. Some examples might include a sprained ankle, a laceration needing stitches, a bout of the flu, a middle-ear infection, or a case of food poisoning. For the most part, this is the way doctors coming out of medical school in America are taught to approach their patients' problems.

This model of care is also currently very popular because it does well with the model of algorithm or treatment-care-guidelines medicine where a computer or kiosk can evaluate a set of symptoms and findings and generate an immediate short-term fix, which can be immediately implemented by a prescribed pill, for example. This model can easily be delegated to implementers with only limited skill and experience, and this dramatically reduces the cost of care and the time and manpower required to perform it. Some are now referring to this as "cookbook medicine."

Traditional, modern-day Western medicine has also fostered the specialty system whereby practitioners become more and more subspecialized and focus on a limited area of expertise. Think of the endocrinologist who has subspecialized to become the diabetologist or the ophthalmologist who has narrowed her focus to become the retinal specialist. The specialists of today literally know more and more about less and less! This subspecialization model makes the prospect of considering the individual as a complete biological system almost impossible.

This approach does not serve the individual suffering from chronic multisystem disease, and it does not lend itself to maintaining the wellness of the "not sick" population.

The failure of this Western model to deal with many chronically ill individuals has led to the emergence of a whole new model of care that focuses on the entire individual and the unique biological system that makes up each person. Disorders of this complex biological system are the fundamental causes of the various symptoms, episodes, and sicknesses that feed into the Western model. This newer model goes by a number of names, such as integrative, holistic, functional, complementary, and alternative. This approach to care does not succeed in the single-episode approach but requires an on-going program of care that addresses the many facets of disturbance to the ideal biological system's function. It requires many small steps rather than a simple, single magic-pill solution. This new model typically requires significant willingness on the part of the patient to become aware of the many factors that lead to disturbances of our biology, which cause disease and premature aging. More importantly, it requires that each individual commit to taking the many steps required to restore the ideal biological system so they can achieve real and sustained wellness.

This new-wellness approach allows each individual to become and feel as well as he or she desires. If you decide you are OK with how you feel and don't want to change anything you're doing, that's fine. It is quite unlikely, however, that a pill is going to be able to, over the long run, restore the biological system in a way that leads to real health and wellness. I don't argue that this would be nice; I just have not found it to be realistic. I don't believe that there is a magic pill. In fact, as the list of synthetic drugs gets longer, the number of adverse interactions tends to rise exponentially, and our fragile chemical-detoxification mechanisms quickly become overburdened. Often, the cure becomes worse than the disease.

It is human nature to desire a quick fix. How often do you hear or read the words "feel better fast" when viewing health-care marketing? This may not always be achievable even with Western medicine. People are accustomed to the fact the chemotherapy used to resolve their cancers may at first make them feel much worse. In fact, we all know that in some cases the treatment can actually kill. So, too, regressive healing may occur in integrative medicine. This means that sometimes a person actually feels worse even as his or her biological system is returning to a more normal state. This is often seen when the process of healing is implemented too quickly or too aggressively.

Fortunately, this is typically short lived, and there are often steps to reduce or reverse the situation.

Some argue that the new integrative medicine is not evidence based. This is completely false. One can argue that there is as much, or more, basic science-based evidence around most of the tenets of integrative medicine as there is in Western medicine. Actually, Western medicine's fixation on the single-agent, randomized, double-blind, placebo-controlled, crossover study lends itself well to the episodic-care model but often does not readily apply to the holistic, functional, and integrative model. It's like trying to compare apples to oranges. It is a completely different paradigm and philosophy.

Over the span of my time in health care, I have been very fortunate to see a steady migration on the part of many providers, and of medicine as a whole, in the direction of a more holistic, functional, systems-biology approach. The transition has been life changing for my patients and for me. I hope you will take the time to become more familiar with this approach to real health and wellness. This handbook is not intended to be a complete presentation of all the many interventions that can, and in most cases should, be used to overcome the chronic diseases of the twenty-first century. In the chapters that follow, I will present the major obstacles to achieving true health and wellness. I will review how these obstacles actually cause the damage that leads to disease and chronic symptoms. I use my mnemonic—*got to shine*—as a catchy, all-inclusive way to remember the main topics of diagnosis and treatment that must be covered along the way. I will mention a variety of treatment principles, but it is not my intention to present a vitamin-by-vitamin, herb-by-herb, hormone-by-hormone, how-to description of health recovery. I encourage the reader who feels that he or she suffers with the conditions I lay out in this handbook to engage the services of a caring, knowledgeable, and committed health-care provider. Select a healer who can play the role of mentor, coach, guide, cheerleader, and yes, at times, prescriber to help you navigate this complex and sometimes confusing pathway to true health and sustained wellness. I am personally passionate and motivated to help people recover and keep real and lasting health in order to live joyful, productive, and active lives.

CHAPTER 2

My Transformation into Integrative Medicine

am the son of a research chemist. I grew up hearing about the latest process to build the world's greatest rocket fuel, the best house paint, or the newest and best synthetic fabric. My dad was the embodiment of the saying, "Better living through chemistry." I actually enjoyed and excelled in my studies in chemistry, especially biochemistry. Mathematics and physics were always favorite subjects as well. Almost of equal interest and ease for me was the study of biology. My eighth-grade biology teacher, William Batey, went way beyond simply teaching his students the laws of biology. He taught us to think and reason about the fascinating intricacies of the life-science world. I don't know how many of Batey's students ended up in the medical field, but I can guarantee you it was way more than a few.

I consistently scored at the top of my class at the University of Texas while majoring in bioengineering and, later, zoology. I graduated with the highest honors. It was an easy choice to pursue a career in medicine, given my aptitude for the basic sciences coupled with my desire to serve my fellow humans. Being a second-generation Eagle Scout helped me learn early on about responsibility, hard work, and citizenship.

For me, deciding to become a surgeon was a fairly easy decision. I have always enjoyed working with my hands, especially small and intricate projects like model building. Choosing to become a head-and-neck/ENT surgeon was also not much of a struggle, as I was drawn to the immensely complex anatomy of that region that houses our unique cosmetic facial features and our complex special senses, not to mention the seemingly countless arteries, nerves, muscles, and other fascinating structures. I was also drawn to the fact in that specialty I could care for adults and children with almost equal frequency. But before I became a head-and-neck surgeon, I was a general physician. I was fortunate to complete my internship year as a general rotating internship. This exposed me to pediatrics, general internal medicine, cardiology, gastroenterology, oncology, and pulmonology. I was similarly blessed to spend my first year of residency as a rotating surgeon and spent time in neurosurgery, oral surgery, plastic surgery, and general surgery. Combining this exposure with the continuing responsibility of manning the emergency department and the acute minor-illness clinic gave me a very well-rounded background as a general practitioner before settling into the head-and-neck/ENT specialty.

Most people don't realize that the ENT/head-and-neck specialty is only about 30–40 percent surgery with 60–70 percent of the experience dealing with the diagnosis and treatment of medical conditions. It is true that as an ENT doctor most of my patients came to me with symptoms of the head and neck, but it was actually the rare patient that only had symptoms confined to that region. While it was gratifying to diagnose and cure an isolated condition like a nosebleed, tonsillitis, or a middle-ear infection, I was always greatly intrigued by the diagnostic dilemmas.

After a gratifying career of nine years as a young US Army medical-corps officer, which allowed my wife and me to see some beautiful places, including three years in western Europe, we chose to settle in the beautiful San Luis valley of Southern Colorado. The Valley, as it is usually called by locals, is known as the "Land of Cool Sunshine" and the "Land of Little Rain." It is an arid plain that stretches between the majestic Sangre de Cristo mountains to the east and the equally grand San Juan mountains to the west. The upper Rio Grande runs right through the heart of the valley. Even though the SLV is a geographically beautiful place, there are hidden dangers beneath the surface. At one point centuries ago, the plain of the San Luis valley had been a very large inland lake. The geology of the valley floor is made up of porous layers of sandy soil, and over time, the lake level fell until all that remained was a huge subterranean aquifer known as the San Luis valley aquifer. The valley has been known for years as a fertile agricultural region with potatoes being one of the principle crops. Since there is not enough rain to support most crops, the farmers depend on sprinkler irrigation from water wells to grow the crops. Many of the crops grown in the valley require substantial amounts of synthetic fertilizers, pesticides, fungicides, herbicides, and defoliants for maximal yields. Over the years, literally tons of petroleum-based chemicals have been sprayed over the valley, and subsequently, they have percolated down into the subterranean aquifer, which just happens to be the drinking-water source for thousands of valley residents. At the same time, an active mining industry is occurring in the mountains that surround the valley. Mine-related chemicals and toxic-heavy metals like cadmium and arsenic have drained incessantly down into the rivers and streams only to gradually percolate in with the rest of the SLV aquifer.

Sure enough, when individuals are exposed to a steady diet of drinking water containing these sorts of ingredients, the results aren't uniformly beneficial. Now, I will grant you that some folks had no problems whatsoever; however, I began to see others suffering from a myriad of chronic environmental-induced illnesses. The sickest of the sick were those individuals who had additional high levels of exposure, such as hair dressers, house cleaners, farmers, diesel mechanics, and the like. Since I had a real interest in these individuals, I started to develop a reputation in my local area as someone who was willing to try to help. I tried all the tricks and tools that conventional medicine had to offer. All of the modern medical knowledge I had received at the University of Texas Southwestern Medical School in Dallas and top-level military medical training had left me incompletely prepared for these chronic diseases. Some of my patients would travel to the ivory towers of Western medicine in nearby major cities. They usually didn't have the answers either. In fact, they would typically come back with the same impressions and treatment recommendations that I had initially concluded but only after relieving the patient of a few thousand dollars.

Out of sheer frustration, I started to search for answers for these patients' desperate circumstances. My quest for answers to these clinical dilemmas led directly into the principles of integrative functional medicine. This requires me to inject a brief comment about the proper title for this new paradigm in health care. Those of us practicing this type of medicine always struggle with what to call it. Up until now, no single, all-inclusive name has emerged. Some use the term "alternative," which stresses the fact that it offers a different—alternate—approach to traditional medicine. Some like the term "functional" as it conveys the understanding that this approach to healing places emphasis on the function of the body's cells, tissues, and organs as a total-body system with a complicated interplay of all the functioning systems. Others prefer the term "holistic," which stresses the whole-body approach to these disease processes in contrast to the individual symptom-problem approach or specialist approach so common with traditional medicine. Rounding out the list are synonyms like complementary, personalized, bioindividualized, and unfortunately, pejorative terms like experimental, nonstandard, and unproven. I personally like the term "integrative," which to me emphasizes that while I embrace this holistic, functional, bioindividualized, alternative approach, at the same time, I retain the many tools in the toolbox of modern-day, conventional Western medicine. Yes, there are plenty of examples when

Western medicine still has what I think is the best answer for a given clinical problem or situation.

What about the concept of standard medical care or the so-called standard of care so often thrown about in the malpractice legal arena? Over the years, I have had plenty of opportunities to chuckle at the times that new, experimental and therefore not standard treatments and techniques have rather quickly become standard and widely embraced. I have also noted with amused interest the many once standard treatments and techniques that have fallen out of favor and sometimes condemned by the established medical authorities. I have not been as amused to consider that one can often follow the money stream to understand which new treatments are embraced or rejected!

There are those who equate integrative medicine with a nonscientific, anecdotal approach to care. Nothing could be further from the truth. The ranks of providers in this growing sphere of healing arts and sciences are filled with many sharp-minded, innovative, conscientious, compassionate healers and scientists performing and publishing state-of-the-art basic science and clinical research. In my observations over four decades of holistic, bioindividualized, integrative medicine, I have witnessed a gradual migration from traditional, prescription-based medicine. The informed public is demanding it.

> It must be considered that there is nothing more difficult to carry out nor more doubtful of success nor more dangerous to handle than to initiate a new order of things; for the reformer has enemies in all those who profit by the old order and only lukewarm defenders in all those who would profit by the new order; this lukewarmness arising partly from the incredulity of mankind who does not truly believe in anything new until they actually have experience of it.
>
> —Niccolo Machiavelli (1469 1527)

Today, I come armed with two toolboxes. One is the toolbox of traditional, episode-based, problem-based, symptom-based, specialist-based, drug-based Western medicine. The other is the new- and rapidly expanding toolbox of the integrative-medical world. I am now much more prepared to assist my patients to pursue a course that restores health and well-being by restoring natural pathways and enabling the body's own inherent healing abilities. My practice today, in a sense, is a return to my early roots as a chemist, mathematician, biologist, and humanist. I now know that I must consider the patient as a very complex and unique whole system. Success requires that the genetic, energetic, social, psychological, chemical, biological, physical, infective, traumatic, spiritual, and environmental factors must all be considered and dealt with as they all contribute to the state of wellness of each one of us.

I want to go on record with my thoughts regarding medical education and the quality of one's abilities as a practitioner of the healing arts. When I was in medical school, we had an expression. What do you call the guy at the bottom of his medical-school graduating class? The answer: Doctor. We used to joke about it, but the point is that having a credential behind your name is not the whole story. An individual's ability to acquire, process, and implement information must always be taken into consideration. It is also critical to consider how conscientious the individual is at staying up with the constant flow of new knowledge. I was blessed to graduate near the top of my class in high school (4th of 650), summa cum laude/Phi Beta Kappa at university, and top 10 percent class rank—Alpha Omega Alpha—in medical school.

Authorities say that the base of scientific and medical knowledge doubles every three years. This may be a bit of an exaggeration even though there is plenty of evidence to support this. I can only say that my knowledge base today bears little resemblance to the knowledge base I took with me the day I left medical school in the seventies. That fund of knowledge was again different than when I initially passed my otolaryngology board examination in the eighties. Unlike most of my head-and-neck/ENT colleagues, I was required to sit for the otolaryngology board recertification examination in 2007. Currently, the American Board of Otolaryngology does not require recertification. I was obliged to complete the American Board of Otolaryngology's recertification program as a condition for Texas relicensure in 2007. I initially was awarded a license to practice medicine after graduating from UT Southwestern medical school in 1978. Since I did not practice in Texas for a period of twenty-nine years, even though I was continuously practicing medicine in the US Army, Colorado, and New Mexico, I chose to forego the not-inconsequential expense of maintaining a Texas license for all those years. When I chose to return to Texas to practice in 2007, I learned that Texas required that I be recertified by the American Board of Otolaryngology. After a six-month period of almost constant literature review and study, I passed on the first try, even though the body of knowledge didn't have much similarity to what I studied for my first board exam in the early eighties.

When you think about it, it makes perfect sense. Over the years, the new discoveries of proteins, enzymes, hormones, inflammatory mediators, germs, viruses, drugs, treatment modalities, testing modalities, and medical devices will absolutely blow you away. Entire new disciplines emerge. Think about surgical robotics or liquid chromatography or rapid gene sequencing. The list goes on and on. What differentiates an older, experienced healer from a young and inexperienced one is the ability to view present-day knowledge through the lens of prior knowledge and experience. If there is one thing I have learned in my decades of work as a healer, it is that there is more than one way to skin a cat. You are less likely to hear a young doctor say this. For them, there is the confident attitude that there is only one way to do something—the way he or she was taught in medical school. Of course, I'm over generalizing to press a point. Unfortunately, some older practitioners do not make the commitment to keep up with the exponential growth of new medical knowledge. I do run into doctors that treat their patients essentially the same way they did when they finished medical school or residency. This is a shame.

When it comes to integrative—or functional, holistic, alternative, complementary—medicine, there is not one unified body of certification of that knowledge base. There are, in fact, many. For me personally, my formal education in integrative medicine has been from a wide variety of sources. I cannot overemphasize from the outset the value of just plain, old experience. The more times you see and deal with a problem or situation the better you learn to handle it. This is especially true if you are honest enough to ask yourself, "Is there a better way I could have done this?" I have learned volumes from exposure to organizations like the American Association of Otolaryngic Allergy, the Pan American Allergy Society, the American Academy of Environmental Medicine, and the American Academy of Anti-Aging and Regenerative Medicine. I have read literally thousands of articles and listened to hundreds of presentations from hundreds of experts. Some are physicians, but many are not. Today's integrative medicine is a discipline with healthy contributions from basic scientists, chiropractors, nutritionists, naturopaths, osteopaths, acupuncturists, counselors, herbalists, homeopaths, physicians, and individuals from many other backgrounds as well. One important caveat—don't believe everything you read! Especially now with the Internet, there is plenty of information posted by those who know just enough to be dangerous. As I acquire new knowledge, I always pass it through the filter of prior knowledge and experience. Honestly, a lot of new knowledge doesn't make the cut and must be thrown out. I caution everyone not to fall into the trap of knowing just enough to be dangerous.

As important as the knowledge and experience is to being a successful healer, it is equally important to consider an individual's ethics, morals, motivations, empathy, and compassion. These characteristics, which often translate into bedside manner, are critical in determining one's ability to be a successful practitioner of the healing arts. This is especially true when the care plan requires a significant "buy in" on the part of the patient. You have to be able to express a certain amount of passion and belief in your message if you ever expect folks to follow your advice, which at times may be quite difficult and undesirable. I don't know of any shortcut to assessing this in any given provider. It is an individual assessment of character between two people. Certainly actions speak louder than words here, and word-of-mouth reviews are a critical indicator.

I have developed a mnemonic to cover the different areas that I must address as I guide a patient toward a condition of real health and true wellness. That mnemonic is *got to shine*. The *g* stands for genetics, the *t* for toxins, the *s* for stress and sleep, the *h* for hormones, the *i* for injury, infection, and inflammation, the *n* for nourishment, and the *e* is for exercise. This serves me well as I go through in my mind the steps in the journey that I must help my patient take in order to arrive at the finish line of ultimate wellness. Needless to say, each one of us has a different relative importance regarding these various problem areas.

I have found that most of us are looking for a quick fix or a miracle pill when it comes to achieving our wellness goals. Sad to say, the times that this is actually possible are few and far between. The functional and integrative approach to health and wellness requires real acceptance and cooperation from the patient because, usually, significant changes in habits, lifestyles, diets, and even interpersonal relationships may be required to achieve complete success. This can be difficult at times. I have found, too, that each individual must strike a balance between changes he or she is willing to make and the degree of symptom relief and restoration of normal function he or she desires to achieve. I often tell patients that I can help them feel as well as they want to feel; the choice is theirs to make.

My transformation into integrative medicine has been a very rewarding evolution toward becoming a wellness detective. I don't have all the answers. No one does. I do have a passion to find all the answers that I can for my patients. This requires me to harness all the scientific knowledge and experience that I can acquire if I am going to be successful in my endeavors. I am required to be a student, teacher, coach, nutritionist, dietician, and cheerleader as well as a doctor. I possess a strong religious faith that comforts me to humbly know that it is not by my own actions and abilities that patients may recover. I rely on God's Spirit constantly to be my guide, support, and strength.

In the pages that follow, I hope to give you a bit of an understanding of the nature of the complex process that I use as an integrative healer. My strong tendency is never to give up on a patient's problems, no matter how complex or seemingly insurmountable they may seem. You don't last very long in this field of health-care delivery if you get easily frustrated or defeated. Now join me as we dive a little deeper into the detective work.

I am going to use the *got to shine* outline as I go through the basics of my approach to healing and wellness as it is the system I use daily in the office.

CHAPTER 3

Genetics: Nature versus Nurture

ommon sense tells us that children, as well as young animals, bear certain features in common with their parents. For as long as humanity has left written records, people have documented the tendency of various traits to pass from generation to generation. The Austrian monk Gregor Mendel performed experiments on pea plants in the 1850s to work out some of the basic principles of this transmission mechanism. Later, in the 1950s, Watson and Crick first described the structure of DNA, which we now know are the molecules that make up the blueprints of our biological makeup—our chromosomes.

It has been recognized for years that certain disorders are passed from parent to child in a predictable way. Examples like sickle-cell anemia, cystic fibrosis, hemophilia, and muscular dystrophy have been recognized by the medical community for years. Some years ago, we developed techniques to visualize the exact nature of the forty-six chromosomes (karyotype analysis) that make us who we are. Twenty-three come from our biological mothers, and twenty-three come from our biological fathers. This ability allowed us to understand many other different inherited conditions like Down syndrome/trisomy 21 and Turner's syndrome, which is a chromosome-deletion condition.

Chromosomes, Genes, and Mutations

We know that our chromosomes, which are made up of long strands of DNA molecules, are arranged into groups known as genes. In the early years of this century, scientists perfected the process that allows them to determine the sequence of our DNA and therefore the sequence of all our genes. This project, known as the Human

Genome Project, was an incredible example of modern science's ability to totally transform our way of thinking about biology, health, and wellness. We have learned that our chromosomes are made up of about six billion base pairs (A, T, C, and G). Three billion each are from mom and dad. We also know that the chromosomes in turn provide the recipe for our abilities to make between twenty-two and twenty-three thousand different, unique human proteins that make us who we are. These proteins are for structure, signaling and communication, recognition, chemical-reaction facilitation (enzymes), and a variety of other special functions. A great number of these unique proteins have been identified, their amino-acid sequence determined, and their purposes have been realized. Each week, new proteins are described, and fairly soon, we will have worked out the nature of all of them. Actually, only about 2 percent of our six billion base pairs is responsible for coding our human proteins. The purpose and function of the other 98 percent is the topic of ongoing research.

There are variations in the DNA base sequences known as SNPs, single-nucleotide polymorphisms, which some people refer to as mutations. It is actually more accurate to consider these to be gene variants even though most of them started as a single mutation that occurred in the distant past from the genes of one of our forefathers or foremothers and subsequently passed down from generation to generation. SNPs are by convention either plus (+) or minus (-). The (-) is often referred to as the wild type. It is usually the type possessed by the majority of the population. The (+) is the variant of the wild type. We normally inherit two copies—again one from mom and one from dad. This creates a situation where we can possess two (-) genes. This is a condition known as homozygous for wild type. If we inherit one (-) and one (+), this is termed the heterozygous condition. Finally, if we inherit (+) (+), we are said to be homozygous for the SNP in question, (double +).

The reason this is so important has to do with the fact alterations of our DNA base sequences associated with these gene-variant SNPs can cause our protein-making machinery to produce an altered protein that may differ significantly from the protein that is made from the wild-type gene. This is a result of an amino-acid substitution, amino acids being the building blocks of our proteins. Depending on the role of the specific protein, these amino-acid substitutions can have a profound effect on our characteristics and our health. We know that everyone possesses hundreds, if not thousands, of different SNP gene-variant mutations. No one, except, in theory, identical twins, has the same combination as anyone else. We really are unique.

If the protein is an enzyme, this alteration can significantly change the protein's enzymatic function. Enzymes enable our metabolic pathways to operate normally by enabling reactions to occur between chemicals that would not occur spontaneously. When one of our enzyme proteins is altered due to SNP gene variance and its associated amino-acid substitution, the metabolic pathway involved can be blocked, or in some cases enhanced, to a greater or lesser degree. In each one of us, there are many examples of these metabolic pathway alterations caused by SNP-induced enzyme variation.

Epigenetics—The Factors Turning Genes On and Off

By themselves, the genes do not necessarily influence our makeup. It is only to the extent that the recipe of each gene is used to build the specific protein that it is programmed to make. Our genes are not making all of our proteins all of the time. There is a very complex system by which the cells know which genes to turn on in order to make proteins at any given point in time. This control process of turning genes on and off is referred to as epigenetics. There are many different factors both from within and without our bodies that affects epigenetics. This is one of the reasons that the debate about the difference between nature—our genes—and nurture—our environments—comes about. Our genes dictate the kinds of proteins we can make, but our environments can control when and which and how much of each protein we make in any cell at any point in time.

Epigenetics is controlled by diet, vitamin status, external toxins, hormones, infections, inflammation, exercise, sleep, age and maturity, our nutritional statuses, and a number of other factors that interact in a complex web. It is for this reason that there is so much argument as to which factor, nature or nurture, is most important. I think clearly both are extremely important.

Currently, as of 2015, there is not much that we can do to change our genes. This is actually starting to change as we learn the techniques of gene alteration, or genetic engineering. Some of this is occurring in the background and may not be desirable. This is part of the argument about genetically modified foods. Some say that they may actually be causing alterations of our genes as we consume them. There is evidence that suggests that certain infections, like viruses, can actually alter our genes as well.

We certainly now know that our gene expression, which proteins are made when, are dramatically altered by many factors that we are exposed to each and every day. In fact, the nature of these exposures is changing at an astounding rate. Think of the monumental number of new synthetic chemicals and the tons of chemicals added to our world each year. Think also of the many physical factors like electromagnetic radiation associated with computers, cell phones, Wi-Fi systems, power lines, and microwave towers. Most of these are not researched, and the nature of their effects on our genes and epigenetics is incompletely understood. Others have been extensively studied, and many have been shown to have profound negative effects on our biological systems and may also have profound negative effects on our health and wellness.

Modern Gene Assessment and Determination of SNP Gene Variants

In my practice, I am able to order a test that uses a saliva sample to sequence a portion of the genes of an individual. This lets me know the status, wild type v. variant, of 825 different gene variants that code for important proteins and enzymes needed by our bodies for our metabolic pathways to function normally. This information is currently available for less than two-hundred dollars. As time passes, the number of genes tested will increase, and the cost will diminish. With further research and experience, we will be better able to predict diseases and, more importantly, intervene to bypass the metabolic blocks associated with the various gene variants.

Now we use the information from the gene results in two main ways. The first way is based on gene-association studies. This line of research depends on the study, which often requires computer data processing, to compare large numbers of different individual's genes against their individual traits and tendencies for various conditions and diseases. This statistical exercise can provide risk assessment, predictive data that can often be helpful in preventing or at least allowing early detection of certain conditions. As the number of different individual data points grows, this information will become more accurate and useful.

The second way that gene-variant data is helpful is by understanding the role of each protein and enzyme within the individual. In the case of an enzyme, the presence of a gene variant coding for that enzyme may result in an amino-acid substitution that may alter the ability of that enzyme to facilitate a chemical reaction in a metabolic pathway. The altered enzyme may cause the reaction of facilitating a slower occurrence (down regulation) or a faster one (up regulation). This is compared to the wild type or native enzyme. In some instances, the altered enzyme might not function at all in its intended role of facilitating a chemical reaction. If the metabolic pathway is needed for energy, less energy may be the result. If the metabolic pathway produces a critical brain chemical, like serotonin, an imbalance may result with obvious effects on mood, sleep, and nerve function. If the metabolic pathway is used to break down a chemical, like caffeine, an intolerance might be the outcome. There are hundreds of examples. As we have more experience, our recommendations will only get better.

The fields of genomics, the study of genes and their effects on health and wellness, and epigenetics and nutragenomics, or the use of the knowledge learned from genes then applied to modify diet and nutrition in a way that gets around the various barriers to the metabolic pathways, are in their infancies. We have only about ten years of experience with this fascinating way to approach our health and wellness in this bioindividualized way. Our way of healing individuals is going to change in exciting and very dramatic ways as this science rapidly emerges.

It is exciting that President Obama recently proposed in early 2015 his precision-medicine initiative to spend 215 million dollars to study the genome results of one-million Americans as a way to rapidly advance clinically useful research. I am personally committed to remain on the cutting edge of this new science that I know is going to bring revolutionary change in the very near future. In my practice today, we assess, evaluate, and develop treatment recommendations based on patient's individual gene-variant results routinely.

CHAPTER 4

Toxins: Are We Slowly Killing Ourselves?

People have always been exposed to environmental toxins. They are not new. Think of our ancient ancestors who might have tried to eat an appetizing yet poisonous berry or mushroom. Think of the times they might have breathed air contaminated with wood smoke in a cave dwelling or the times they may have tried to drink water contaminated with harmful minerals, germs, or parasites. The point here is that our bodies have always possessed elegant systems that God gave us to deal with these various harmful toxins or poisons in our environments so that we could survive them. These systems, however, were designed to deal with relatively low levels of toxic exposures. So what has changed?

Public-health research is indicating that we are experiencing an explosion in the incidence of a number of different chronic health conditions that are related to ongoing inflammation within our bodies. We have long understood that inflammation caused by our immune system is one of the most important ways that we deal with external toxins. Inflammation that is vital for protection is a double-edged sword. Inflammation is not able to discriminate what it strikes. In other words, when our bodies launch inflammation against a foreign toxin or invader, our own cells and tissues get hit in the crossfire. This is sometimes called the innocent-bystander effect.

Nowadays, especially since the Industrial Revolution, the amount of toxins in the environment has dramatically increased and is continuing to increase by the day. Just look at the air pollution in Beijing, China, that is frequently in the news today. There are thousands of examples, and we hear about new ones constantly. The primitive yet elegant mechanisms that our bodies possess to deal with these harmful environmental exposures were never designed to deal with these amounts of toxin exposure. Each one of us, due to our own unique genetics and epigenetics, have different abilities to inactivate, remove, break down, or otherwise deal with these environmental toxic insults. In other words, some of us are very proficient at dealing with even large amounts of pollution and toxins while others are not proficient at all. This helps to explain why in any population only a fraction of people actually begin to have symptoms, but over time, the number of people affected steadily increases if levels of exposure increase. The most sensitive individuals are the canaries in the coalmine so to speak.

The obvious question becomes, What can be done to remedy the situation? There is an answer, but it is a complex one. It is critical, though, to address it if we are to get a handle on the steadily increasing amount of chronic, inflammation-based diseases that are affecting more and more of our population. Diseases like autism, asthma, diabetes, obesity, cancer, heart disease, Alzheimer's disease, autoimmune syndromes, mood disorders, migraine headaches, allergies, irritable bowel syndrome, and chronic fatigue are but a few of the disorders that are increasing in the population and appear to have ties to environmental triggers. No one is immune. It affects men, women, children, the young, and the old. Let's try to explore what we can do individually and collectively to deal with the problem of environmental toxins.

Learning to Avoid Environmental Toxin Exposures

I always tell my patients that are showing signs and symptoms of toxic damage that the first thing to do is make every effort to stop the onslaught of toxins entering the body. If your body is not working due to toxic exposure, then by all means, stop exposing it to more toxins. Although this might seem simple, it is actually almost impossible to accomplish—although there are definite steps we can take. Studies now show that every baby born in America who is tested has measurable levels of a significant number of foreign chemicals known to be associated with harmful effects. Tests of umbilical cord blood will register positive for environmental toxins.

Since environmental toxins enter our bodies through the air we breathe, the liquids we drink, the food we eat, and the substances that we put on our skin, these are the sources that we need to consider.

In Quest of Safe Food

I am often asked which is the best beverage to drink. The answer is really simple: clean water and lots of it! Most people don't drink nearly enough. Drinking water needs to be as free as possible of plastic residues, chemicals like chlorine and fluorine, pesticides and fertilizers, residues of drugs, and so forth. Nowadays, as more and more waste water is being recycled back into the drinking water supply, the problem is growing because the systems in place to accomplish the recycling are not able to remove 100 percent of all chemicals. Drinking water that is subjected to reverse osmosis is a good step. So too is drinking water from nonplastic containers. Distilling water removes many, but not all, toxins. Mountain spring water is usually a very good source of water. The amount of fluid we should drink daily varies, but a good rule of thumb is to drink a half ounce of fluid—all beverages consumed—for each pound of body weight. Some folks like the eight-by-eight rule, eight glasses of eight ounces, which is an easy to remember rule for adults. Again, most of us need to drink quite a bit more clean water each day. Water is vital for normal metabolic and kidney function.

What about food? Specific diet recommendations to assist with detoxification are beyond the scope of what I plan to cover in this brief introduction, but some general comments about safe food are definitely in order. I encourage my patients to eat as organically as they can afford. Today, organic food is still more expensive, although this is starting to change. I tell my patients to eat real food or food that their great, great grandmother would recognize as food. This eliminates most processed foods. Typically, if you shop around the border of the grocery store, you tend to find more fresh food as opposed to processed food. I also tell my patients to read food labels and try to avoid foods with lots of food additives, like artificial colorings, artificial flavorings, preservatives, binders, stabilizers, texturizers, etc. Typically, the shorter the list of added ingredients the better. Green, leafy vegetables tend to be rich in nutrients as are dark-red and blue fruits like blueberries, cranberries, blackberries, currants, goji, and noni berries. I suggest that my patients eat plenty of vegetables from all the colors of the rainbow. If you know you don't tolerate a food, it is always best to avoid it. I recommend avoidance of refined sugars and starches almost always. I encourage sticking with heathy fats like coconut oil, olive oil, and avocado oil and avoiding trans fats and hydrogenated fats often found in fast food. I encourage emphasizing omega-3 fatty acids, as in fish and flax seed, while underemphasizing vegetable oils. It is very important to thoroughly wash fruits and vegetables in order to remove as much of any chemical residue as possible. There are often lots of nutrients and useful fiber in the skins of many fruits and vegetables, but we don't want any chemicals that might have been applied during production. We are beginning to understand that genetically modified foods may be problematic. Many GMO foods are made to be Roundup ready, which means they have been modified to resist the herbicidal effects of glyphosate—the generic name for Roundup. Growers can then use glyphosate aggressively to kill out undesirable weeds. They have even found that glyphosate can be useful in drying out certain crops as they approach harvest time. The amount of glyphosate being applied to our food supply continues to rise as weeds are becoming more and more resistant to it. Science is showing that there are plenty of harmful effects associated with glyphosate consumption by humans. This video is a useful resource on the hazards of glyphosate: www.vimeo.com/115304371.

Don't Forget the Skin

Don't overlook the skin as a route for harmful and toxic chemicals into our bodies. The review process for cosmetics leaves much to be desired in terms of ingredient safety. Many people have obvious symptoms of intolerance, such as rashes, burning, or headache, but often, the harmful effects are only seen after prolonged exposure. Frequently, two or more harmful chemicals have synergistic toxic effects where symptoms may only occur or be worsened when both ingredients are ingested at the same time. One plus one can equal three in this situation. Watch for deodorants with aluminum, BHA, formaldehyde, parabens, phthalates, propylene glycol, and siloxanes. By far the best way to handle toxins entering our bodies through the skin is to simply avoid them. Learn to read labels of products and become familiar with the list of known bad actors. Please be aware that new ingredients are being made constantly, and frequently, cosmetic manufacturers change ingredients with little or no notification to the consumer. For this reason, it is not unusual to see someone react to a product suddenly that never caused a problem before.

The chemical industry develops new petroleum-based chemicals or modifies known natural chemicals at a staggering and exponential rate. Unfortunately, the groups that are tasked to monitor these new chemicals for safety, including government organizations like the EPA and FDA, are not equipped to keep up with the pace of development that is, of course, largely driven by profit motives of the developers. The lobbying efforts on the part of the manufacturers and developers presents a formidable obstacle to maintaining consumer safety. It is not unusual to see an ingredient declared harmful and therefore unacceptable only months to years after it has been in common usage.

Even the most compulsive efforts to avoid exposure to toxins in the air, food, water, and skin are not at all adequate to stop the onslaught on our bodies. It is important to have at least an elementary understanding of the mechanisms we were born with to detoxify these harmful substances. Our detox mechanisms were never intended to deal with the sheer magnitude of the amount of present-day exposure. Many of the toxic substances, especially the petroleum-based ones, are quite stable and have half-lives lasting years and even decades. Also, many of these chemicals are fat soluble, which means they tend to end up in our fat cells where they can remain for a lifetime while slowly dribbling out into our circulation where their toxic effects are seen in other cells and tissues.

The Role of Detoxification

The detoxification process is a three-phase process for many toxins. The liver and kidneys do the lion's share of the work. In the first step, the body must use a system of specialized protein enzymes to react with specific toxic substances to prepare them for elimination. This often involves converting a substance from a fat-soluble one to a water-soluble one. The cytochrome P450 or CYP system is a sophisticated group of enzymes tasked with the initiation of this conversion. This first phase actually renders the toxic substance more unstable and potentially more dangerous to our own cells and self structures than before. The body tries to quickly apply a second phase that is able to attach a chemical to the activated toxin so that it becomes more water soluble and is easier to eliminate. Phase two includes several different pathways; these include methylation, sulfonation, glucuronidation, and acetylation, which attach specific groups to the activated toxins that then can more easily be eliminated from the body. The third and final step is excretion whereby the more water-soluble toxins can be expelled through urine, bile, sweat, and feces. We now understand that the different steps of this complex process are based on metabolic pathways that are driven by protein enzymes that we possess. Due to genetic variation, SNP/gene mutations, some individuals are much better detoxifiers than others. This helps to explain why in any population of people exposed there are always those who will fall ill the earliest.

Today, with the development of genome testing, we are becoming able to identify in advance those individuals who are at greater risk of diseases associated with toxic exposure or intolerance of specific toxins. This can be helpful when counseling folks on toxin-exposure avoidance. We are also learning that once we are aware of the inherited genomic blocks to normal metabolic function, we find that there are also steps that can often be taken to maximize these detox pathways. It is possible that in the future there may even be ways to alter genes in such a way to improve detox function.

Avoiding toxins takes all of us

As important as it is to know what individual steps can be taken to avoid and reduce the risks of environmental toxin exposure, I believe that we have to do more as a community to clean up the environment. I am not really suggesting a specific solution. There seems to be more lip service than actual results. The statistics on the rate of environmental degradation over the past fifty years are really staggering. It is not something that gets very much air time, since big money really doesn't want us to even know that a problem exists. My only plea is that individuals make a commitment to understand the enormity and critical nature of the problem and begin to take steps toward becoming part of the solution. If you don't do it for yourself, do it for your children and grandchildren. Together, I promise you that we can make a significant difference.

In my integrative-medicine clinic, I help people learn how to best avoid, eliminate, and neutralize these toxins in a way that helps them ultimately achieve true health and wellness and maintain it for the long haul.

CHAPTER 5

Stress and Sleep Disorder: Two Silent Killers

The *s* in *got to shine* stands for stress and sleep. These two really go together as a team in contributing to our poor health. The fact stress makes us sick is common knowledge just as much as the fact we humans do not do well when we are sleep deprived. Only recently has modern science really begun to unravel the mechanisms that account for these common-sense observations. I am going to try to shed some light on these factors, and I am going to take them one by one, even though there is a substantial amount of overlap between them.

The Importance of Learning to Limit and Manage Stress

Let's start with stress. For as long as I've been a doctor, I have always told my patients that they need to learn to deal with stress if they are going to become truly well and stay that way. I had never really understood, until much more recently, just how important this is or what the actual mechanisms are. There is now a very active body of research and scientific study that is working out these mechanisms. Research is connecting stress to almost all inflammation-based, chronic diseases. Heart disease, stroke, hypertension, diabetes, obesity, asthma, autoimmunity, headache, and cancer are just a few of the diseases caused by stress. We are just now understanding how steps to eliminate stress in our lives results in definite, and sometimes dramatic, resolution and prevention of many disorders.

To better understand how this is so, we need to understand a bit more about stress itself. Humans have always had a response to stress. In the past, humans would react to a stressful situation with what's known as the fight-or-flight response. An example of this is when someone is being chased by a lion. This is essentially the same response that triggers an animal stampede. This fight-or-flight or panic response is a very normal physiological series of changes in the body that happens almost instantly when the body's sensors—eyes, ears, nose, and skin—perceive an environmental threat. If the threat is bad enough, a reflex is triggered involving the brain, which then sends signals to the rest of the body. This reflex is designed to allow the body to deal with the threat. The sudden stress response triggers neurons and nerves that release certain chemicals, neurotransmitters, and other signaling molecules, hormones and other circulating mediators, that induce changes like faster heart rate, more rapid breathing, and higher blood pressure. Our senses become much more aware, our muscles are dramatically stronger, and our ability to metabolize sugar for energy speeds up. All good, right?

Sort of. Even though the sudden response to a real environmental threat may be essential to our survival, the problem comes about when these triggering events are part of our everyday routine. When we experience stress responses excessively or when our bodies become stuck in an ongoing state of stress, problems start to be seen. Over time, the effects of the stress response lead to harmful outcomes in the body.

The Role of the Adrenal Gland in Response to Stress

The adrenal gland is sometimes referred to as our stress gland. It is richly supplied with nerves from the brain that, when stimulated, result in a release of adrenalin and noradrenalin, as well as cortisol and other signaling molecules and mediators that mediate the normal stress response and also often contribute directly to disease. There are many other ways, but this is one of the best understood. People sometimes tease that someone or something "really squeezed my adrenals."

Assessment of adrenal function and correction of identified problems is one important way to reverse the harmful effects of ongoing stress. When exposed to chronic stress, the adrenal gland typically undergoes a transition from a condition of adrenal overactivity to ultimately reach a state of deficiency or adrenal fatigue. The treatment varies with the position on this continuum of imbalance.

Just as with environment chemicals, one of the principles of treatment is to remove the sources of stress. As with toxin exposure in today's world, this can be much more easily said than done. Our world today is literally filled with stress-causing environmental stimuli. Have you heard of multitasking? This is a modern-day way of saying excess-stressing. Our modern devices—computers, television, cell phones, stereos, and even electric lighting—have done much to add stress to our existence. Almost everyone admits to too much stress in their routines. Financial stress and relational stress occur nowadays in epidemic amounts. A toxic personal relationship can cause every bit as much disease as a toxic chemical.

I used to glibly tell my patients, "Try to reduce the sources and amounts of stress in your life." I now understand that this is in no way enough. I have become much more intentional in the ways I try to help my patients reduce stress. I can honestly say that this is a process that I cannot adequately achieve on my own. Even though I am exceptionally well trained and aware of the triggers, mechanisms, and techniques for treating stress, the daily management of stress really requires a team approach. Knowledge is power when it comes to stress reduction. But successful stress management is an ongoing life process that can include religious teachers, exercise coaches, life coaches, meditation mentors, counselors, massage therapists, yoga instructors, chiropractors, and many, many others. It must become a part of one's daily routine. The point is to address stress and begin to deal with it. You can't make stress reduction the last thing you deal with. It really needs to occur at the beginning of the wellness process, or you may never see real improvement.

How Sleep Contributes to Our Health and Wellness

Sleep is an amazingly complex problem. For years, we have understood the harmful effects of sleep deprivation. In fact, it is used as a cruel form of torture to manipulate individuals, but I don't really want to go there. I can't tell you how often I hear my patients tell me they got worse or got sick because they weren't getting enough sleep. Sleep is a condition of the body that is used for restoration and recuperation of many bodily processes. It is a complex condition that results from an intricate balance of nervous, hormones, and other signaling molecules needed to orchestrate and induce the type and stages of sleep that are needed for the body to function in an ideal way.

Like with toxins and stress, the modern world is much less conducive to good sleep than in times past. We live in a twenty-four-hour-a-day world. We can access many types of media any minute of the day. Many businesses operate 24/7 now. Shift work and night shifts are ever more commonly seen. Chronic stress is a significant contributor to disrupted and reduced sleep. Airway obstruction, which can cause sleep apnea, is much more common now with the substantial rise in overweight individuals. Increased allergies result in nasal blockage and tonsil enlargement, and both are known to adversely affect sleep.

The use of powerful synthetic drugs to induce sleep may result in short-term benefits, but this frequently only reduces the chances for restoration of the normal biological mechanisms that can lead to sustained, healthy sleep patterns.

Addressing chronic stress is essential to establishing and maintaining normal sleep patterns. Hormones like cortisol, thyroid, estrogen, progesterone, testosterone, melatonin, and oxytocin all play a very important role in sleep. Sleep patterns are set by the brain, and we know that the proper balance of a number of brain chemicals called neurotransmitters is required for sleep to occur in a normal way. The neurotransmitters dopamine, serotonin, epinephrine, and norepinephrine are susceptible to significant metabolic-pathway abnormalities often related to disorders of the methylation cycle and other enzyme-mediated pathways. As in other areas of metabolism, our genome mutations often contribute in a significant way to sleep problems. It is common to see insomnia and other types of sleep disorders cluster in family groups as a result of these genetically inherited tendencies.

Genome testing is often useful to overcome poor sleep. When the nature of the gene-mediated, metabolic-pathway abnormalities is understood, as in the case of other genome-mediated mutations, there are steps that can often be taken to safely and naturally bypass the metabolic blocks and neurotransmitter imbalances without having to resort to powerful and potentially addicting synthetic drugs. I always talk to my patients about normal sleep hygiene. Common sense should tell you not to consume products like caffeine and other stimulants shortly before bedtime. Preparing for bedtime by setting a regular time for sleep devoid of distractions is helpful. Some people sleep better when there is relaxing sound such as soft music or environmental sound like a fan running. Absolute darkness is most consistent with good sleep. The exact amount of sleep needed for ideal health varies from individual to individual. Our sleep needs tend to go down as we age and vary within each of us depending on both internal and external factors.

I have seen many cases over the years where simply helping a patient have consistent, uninterrupted, and adequate sleep resulted in dramatic resolution of many other symptoms and diseases. As with stress management, sleep needs to be addressed early on in treatment.

CHAPTER 6

Hormones: A Harmonious Hormone Symphony Is Required for Ideal Health

Many of the symptoms seen in patients with chronic, inflammation-induced disorders—usually with methylation-cycle abnormalities as one of the root causes—can be explained by various hormone deficiencies, excesses, or imbalances. Attending to the normalization of metabolic pathways, nutrient status, and mitochondrial function often results in substantial restoration of normal hormone function. This is a key to success in recovery. Very often, these blocks to normal metabolic-pathway function result in a broad array of hormone deficiencies and imbalance conditions. Increasing environmental toxin exposure exacerbates these problems. Since restoring normal metabolic pathways is, by necessity, a gradual, step-by-step process, significant symptom improvement can often be achieved much more quickly through the use of a variety of bioidentical hormones, including hypothalamic, pituitary, adrenal, thyroid, pancreatic, ovarian, and testicular. As the biological processes recover and metabolic pathways are restored to more normal function, bioidentical hormone requirements may be reduced or end altogether.

Optimum Hormone Balance Is Like a Symphony

Over the past twenty-five years that I have treated chronic, inflammation-induced illness, I have seen very few cases associated with what I would consider ideal hormone balance. I believe there are a number of reasons that explain my observation. To start with, our system of hormones—along with complex contributions from multiple other signaling molecules, including proteins as well as small molecule signalers—is an extraordinarily complex system. It is not a static system but one that constantly fluxes depending on a great number of factors. I think of it like a masterpiece symphony played by a large orchestra. The analogy is actually quite appropriate. Our hormones, like the music, are constantly changing throughout the days, months, and years of our lives. The various hormones interact with each other in complex ways. For optimum hormone balance, there must be a delicate yet constantly changing harmony. Our hormone requirements constantly change based on our health, age, sex, and nutritional status. Our stress levels and sleep influence hormones as does physical activity, diet, disease, infection, inflammation, and exposure to toxins. In addition to substantial variation in the level of hormones, we are constantly experiencing changes in the quantity and sensitivity of a large number of hormone receptors and molecules called second messengers, which relay hormone messages inside the cells.

Hormones and hormone receptors being unique proteins are each subject to alteration of function due to inherited genome SNP/mutations. We are just now beginning to use genome testing to understand and predict functional hormone disorders. In the future, this understanding and the application of appropriate interventions will only increase to the benefit of patients.

Another reason that so few of my chronically ill patients are in ideal hormone balance results from genetically inherited metabolic disorders, particularly methylation cycle abnormalities. Multiple methylation steps are required in the pathways that lead to the formation of our hormones. The steroid hormones, for example, are synthesized in the mitochondria and smooth endoplasmic reticulum; these are delicate structures inside our cells. They are easily damaged by free radicals that are often elevated when methylation is not progressing optimally. Chronic inflammation as of the autoimmune variety often affects the various hormone-producing glands resulting in cell and tissue injury that adversely affects hormone levels and hormone balance. Many external chemical toxins acquired from the environment contribute to abnormal hormone gland function as well. Chronic infection agents, such as viruses, may infect hormone glands, which also contributes to hormone problems.

The Difference between Normal
Hormone Levels and Optimum Levels

My philosophy of hormone management is what is sometimes called functional endocrinology. Functional endocrinology is hormone management that varies rather significantly from the approach of some traditionally practicing Western endocrinologists.

To show the difference, I need to explain just a little bit about the concept of normal hormone lab values. When a hormone is measured—whether it be a saliva measurement, a blood measurement, or a urine measurement—the resulting value is reported against a reference range. This reference range is an observed range determined by compiling the values of a large group of the population. This generates a range of values from low to high. The normal range is generally based on the numbers within which 95 percent of the population would fall. The range takes into account all individuals, including healthy and less healthy folks, without taking into account any confounding factors that may be in play. In functional endocrinology, hormone values are compared not against the 95 percent distribution range, but they are instead considered in the context of an ideal value or range that takes into account the conditions of the individual patient at the time of the test. In other words, it might be normal for a lady with severe fatigue to have a thyroid level just above the lower limit of normal, but for her condition, it is almost certainly well below the level that is consistent with maximum health and wellness. Functional endocrinology involves adjusting hormone administration based on the optimization of symptoms more than on theoretical and broad normal ranges.

The Role of Hormones in Aging

The aging process is associated with significant, and often dramatic, declines in hormone levels. This varies by hormone but can begin as early as the third decade of life. By age seventy, the levels of some hormones have declined to 10–20 percent of the maximal levels seen in the early twenties. It is a hotly debated topic among healthcare providers treating aging patients as to whether the drop in hormones is a consequence of the aging process. I believe it doesn't matter. Regardless of the answer to this theoretical question, the aging process can be slowed by achieving more youthful hormone levels consistent with younger individuals. This is also frequently associated with marked improvement in overall metabolic and biological function.

Bioidentical Hormones versus Synthetic Hormones

The use of bioidentical hormones, which are exact replicas of the actual human hormones, appear to be the best and safest way to replace and restore hormone function that is consistent with optimum cellular function, optimum health, and optimum wellness. Bioidentical hormones are not subject to patent protection in the same way that synthetic man-made hormones are. This is a key reason that bioidentical hormones have been aggressively opposed by powerful factors within traditional Western medicine. An understanding of symptoms and signs associated with hormone deficiency and excess is often the best way to adjust and balance hormones in order to maximize health and wellness. Lab values can be used to assure that hormone levels and important hormone metabolites are in desirable ranges, but the real fine-tuning comes from comparing how you feel against the hormones you are using. Many of my patients learn to recognize how their bodies respond to the various hormones and how there hormone requirements change based on their day-to-day circumstances. In these individuals, I actually encourage minor self-adjustments to replacement doses in order to maximize symptom improvement.

Many patients, especially those with a history of cancer are quite fearful of the role that hormones may play in worsening or contributing to the recurrence of their cancers. This is perfectly understandable! Often this mind-set has been deeply instilled into their thinking and understanding by well-meaning health-care providers. In fact, many of my patients have been treated with techniques and drugs designed to remove or reduce the actions of various natural human hormones. There is a general climate of concern that hormone replacement may contribute to other adverse health outcomes like blood clots or heart attacks. There have been a number of well-done, large, scientific clinical studies that have looked specifically into these risks and have shown with a high degree of statistical confidence that there is no increased risk with appropriate dosages of bioidentical hormones. The results of similar studies using synthetic man-made hormones instead of bioidenticals has tended to show much more association with adverse and dangerous effects. When you balance the beneficial effects against the low likelihood of risk, the argument in favor of using bioidentical hormone replacement becomes quite compelling.

In my integrative-medical clinic, the use of bioidentical-hormone-replacement therapy after appropriate assessment plays an important role in contributing to true health, sustained wellness, and the reduction of premature aging.

CHAPTER 7

Inflammation, Infection, and Injury: Staying Clear of Friendly Fire

n my *got to shine* mnemonic, the *i* stands for three interrelated causes of disease: inflammation, infection, and injury. Injury can, of course, be due to physical injury, as with a burn, a fall, or a laceration. The ill effects of these are rather easy to imagine and understand. There is another form of injury that is harder to see. This is the form of microscopic injury that occurs at the cellular level. It is a consequence of the other two causes: infection and inflammation.

Inflammation—The Good News/Bad News Story

Understanding inflammation requires a definition of the term and an explanation of why and how it contributes to cellular, tissue, and organ injury and therefore disease. Inflammation is defined as a local tissue response to an infection or injury. It is further defined by its classic hallmarks of redness, pain, swelling, and warmth. Inflammation is sometimes only detected by microscopic examination or laboratory identification, although it is usually suspected from symptoms or signs in the patient. Inflammation is a complex cascade of events generated by our body's immune system. To some people, it is surprising to learn that inflammation is actually a critical requirement for life. It is necessary to eliminate, destroy, inactivate, or isolate potentially harmful external agents from the body. Often, these are infection-causing agents like viruses, bacteria, yeasts, fungi, and parasites. If it were not for the immune system and the inflammation that it generates, we would die and die quickly.

The immune system and the inflammatory process that it generates are incredibly complex and highly advanced systems of protection. Unraveling the mystery of these amazing systems is still far from complete. The level of our understanding, and therefore our ability to manipulate and alter the course, is increasing almost at an exponential rate.

Appreciating the Complexity of the Immune System

Humans are made up of about two hundred different types of cells. Consider the differences between neurons in the brain, white blood cells, bone cells, skin cells, liver cells, kidney cells, and heart-muscle cells to list but a few. Then think about the fact all these cells contain the same genetic blueprint—the blueprint that was created when our parents' sperm and egg combined to become a complete fertilized egg cell at our conceptions. You may ask what then causes these cells to look and act so differently. The difference is due to epigenetics. Epigenetics is the phenomenon that determines and controls which of our twenty-two thousand protein-making genes are turned on or off in any given cell at any given time. This ability to turn on and off genes is not a yes/no proposition, but it also has the ability to tell how much a gene should be turned on or off. This epigenetic process is again amazingly complex and subject to a vast number of different influences and regulatory signals—some internal and some external. The immune system is comprised of probably the widest variety of different types of cells of any system in the body. There are at least twenty different cell types. As science develops, new ways to subclassify these cells makes their numbers increase. In fact, the system possesses the capability of frequently inducing cells to morph into new types on command. Some cells circulate throughout the body in the blood vessels, lymph vessels, and capillaries, and other cells are fixed within tissues. Still others are capable of migrating between the circulatory system and the tissues.

These various cells, in turn, are capable of making an astounding array of protein molecules as directed by our individual protein-coding genes and the various epigenetic signals turning those genes on and off. The number of proteins that have been identified and described as playing a role in this system already numbers in the hundreds, and the list grows rapidly. These proteins are used by the system as structural proteins for the cells themselves, but they can also be used as cell receptor proteins, circulating signaling proteins, surveillance proteins, and effector proteins. Categories of these proteins include antibodies, cytokines, lymphokines, interleukins, complement, trophic factors, and catalytic enzymes.

The human immune system is quite advanced in comparison to more simple forms of life that also possess primitive systems of immunity. Human immunity is broadly divided into the innate (already present) and acquired or adaptive (that which must develop on demand) arms of the system. Innate immunity is the more primitive part of the system. This is typically the first part of the system to jump into action at the earliest arrival of a foreign invader. At essentially the same time, the adaptive immune system also joins the fight, although there is typically a time lag before the system becomes completely operational. The analogy to a military defense system is quite appropriate. There are the local defense teams that remain at the ready to respond immediately to threat until the main army can arrive and provide powerful reinforcements.

Autoimmunity—Allergy to Self

Early in the process, the system is tasked with monitoring the landscape for threats. Think of this as the early-warning or intelligence arm of the system. This complex system must differentiate friend from foe. Our immune surveillance system is tasked to identify early cancer cells in addition to infection agents. To be successful, this requires that the system be fairly accurate at identifying the enemy early on and not mistake the good guys for the enemy. When the immune system mistakes the good guys as being part of the enemy, it may launch an attack against the body itself. This is one form of autoimmunity.

Once it is determined that a threat exists, the system swings into action. The immune system begins to try to isolate the threat so that it doesn't become widespread. Reinforcements are called in. Cells are tasked, when possible, to engulf or literally eat the attackers, much like in the game Pacman. If they can't be engulfed, then the immune cells try to surround the attackers as best as they can. At this point, the immune cells use a host of effector proteins. Think of these as the actual bullets and artillery shells in the battle. As in a real military conflict, the various effector proteins possess no real ability to judge what they hit. Once they are released, they damage friendly cells and tissues even as they damage, and hopefully eliminate, the foreign attackers. To minimize self-injury, the system tries to keep the effector proteins in as close proximity to the battle as it can. The effector proteins include a number of enzymes that act as catalysts to break down the proteins, fats, and carbohydrate molecules of the invading organisms or cancer cells. Many of these molecules form what are called free radicals or reactive oxygen species (ROS). These free radicals are highly reactive molecules that, like the cue ball on the pool table, tend to alter anything they contact—friend or foe.

So let's suppose we won the battle, and the threat is gone. At this point, it is critical that the body have a mechanism to stop the attack and begin to clean up and rebuild the battlefield. This first requires that the body use a sophisticated system of antioxidant and detox mechanisms to mop up the live shells and land mines still lying around. Actually, the antioxidants and other proteins are tasked with disenabling the various effector proteins so they do not cause further injury to the self. Cells and a variety of signaling proteins are needed to pass the word that the threat is now gone and everyone can go back to what they were doing. A complex process of clearing away the debris and rebuilding then begins. This process can last for years.

Our human immune system actually possesses the ability to remember the nature of the attack, and it maintains the ability to more immediately jump into action if the attacking threat ever recurs. This memory is the principle behind the theory of immunization.

Assessing the immune system

How is immune function assessed? The tools used to assess human immunity have arguably evolved more over the thirty-plus years that I have practiced medicine than any other area—with the possible exception of genetic assessment. Even as our understanding of this immensely complex system has advanced, so too have our methods used to assess it. In medical school, we used the CBC, the serum protein electrophoresis, the erythrocyte sedimentation rate (ESR or sed rate), the differential white blood cell count on the blood smear, and the skin response test. That's all now considered to be from the dark ages. Today, we have very sophisticated techniques to measure the relative and absolute numbers of a whole host of different types of lymphocytes and other white blood cells. We now have the capability of measuring with a high degree of accuracy very minute quantities of a very large number of different proteins and small molecules that participate in the inflammatory response at different levels. We can assess independently different subparts of the immune response. We have sophisticated tools to measure immune antibody proteins directed against an enormous array of different antigenic substances, which is able to stimulate an immune response, both of the self and nonself. We have elegant assays and techniques to measure the function of the different parts of the system in operation at any given time. The question is not how to assess the immune system as much as it is the question of how to assess it in a cost-effective way that results in meaningful therapeutic decision making. I often tell patients that we can spend thousands of dollars testing, yet much of the testing will be of limited value and may not alter in any meaningful way our recommendations for intervention. I absolutely do not believe in testing out of interest alone, and I really object to the whole concept of defensive or CYA testing. However, I will admit that sometimes testing must be undertaken in order to convince the patient or family of the need for certain interventions or actions.

Through the years, I have had the occasion to deal with literally thousands of cases of inflammation. In the early years of my medical practice, I used the tools in the toolbox that I had been given in my traditional medical training to deal with infection. These included surgical techniques, antibiotics, antiseptics, anti-inflammatory agents like steroids and NSAIDs, antihistamines, and immunizations. Most cases improved and resolved without much incident, but there were often undesirable side effects and, of course, the occasional failure. I had been taught how to deal with the undesirable injury associated with autoimmunity with powerful synthetic drugs like prednisone and methotrexate whose purpose was to suppress or disenable the immune system. I always struggled with the rationale behind suppressing the immune system. It always seemed a bit dangerous and extreme to me. It reminds me a little bit of what we used to say as surgeons in training—tongue in cheek, of course—"When in doubt, cut it out." As my experience and my understanding of the systems biology involved in the process continued to rapidly grow along with the realization that there was a whole new realm of treatment options aimed at enabling, rebalancing, and optimizing the various aspects of the system in natural ways, I was able to dramatically improve my outcomes and avoid many of the side effects associated with the synthetic drugs. I started to see fewer failures and fewer side effects.

The Role of the Immune System in Allergy

While we are considering inflammation, I would like to make some comments about allergy and autoimmunity. The immune surveillance aspect of the early-warning part of the immune system is, of course, tasked with differentiation of friend from foe. In the course of this activity, it is not uncommon to identify many examples where the immune system determines that something it encounters is a threat and should therefore be attacked when the substance is actually not a threat. Think of pollen grains, dust, mold spores, or animal dander entering our eyes and noses. When the immune system launches an attack against these harmless external visitors to neutralize them and the resulting release of inflammatory effectors causes injury to our own tissues—histamine release causing itchy eyes, stuffy nose, burning, and sneezing—this is an allergic condition. Also, if the immune system determines that our tissues are foreign and need to be attacked—think of rheumatoid arthritis in the joints or Hashimoto's thyroiditis in the thyroid—the result is injury to self-structures as a result of the in-flammatory attack that the immune system unleashes.

Why do only some of us tend to develop allergies and autoimmunity? Why is the incidence of allergic and autoimmune disease rising so rapidly per capita in the indus-trialized world? Why do some people go through much of their lives without suffering from these conditions only to suddenly develop them at some later point? I think these are really intriguing questions that have their answers in new understandings about the role of our genes, our epigenetics, our nutrients, and the effects of many external environmental agents that we are encountering in larger numbers and larger quantities. As we gain a better understanding of these principles, we will begin to identify ways of restoring normal biological system function that reverse and prevent these chronic, inflammation-induced diseases. I have learned to harness many of these new, more natural, functional, and holistic tools as I help my patients navigate a course back to health and wellness.

Immune System's Role in Infection Control

Most of the discussion of the immune system and inflammation leads back to infec-tion. Infection is, after all, the raison d'être of the immune system in the first place. As we have discussed above, not all inflammation results from infection, even if it is the ultimate purpose of inflammation. The subject of infection could be a whole book unto itself. I'm not going to go to anywhere near that extreme, but there is much use-ful information that I have acquired that with the knowledge of both traditional as well as functional, holistic medicine allows me to present some very useful facts, in my humble opinion.

The list of threats in the infectious-disease world is very long and continues to grow. That growth is largely due to the discovery of new infectious agents but also includes the alarming realization that new infective agents are coming onto the scene all the time. Think of the new strains of flu viruses, Ebola viruses, flesh-eating bacteria, antibiotic-resistant germs, discovery of the prion-causing mad cow disease, various germs associated with Lyme-associated diseases, and so on. Science is racing to keep up with this growing list of threats. We may not be doing such a great job of keeping up.

In my practice over the years, it has been my experience that much of the disease associated with infection actually results from a deficient, imbalanced, overactive, or otherwise impaired immune system. When I was in medical school, we learned about a handful of named immune-deficiency syndromes and a catch-all known as combined immune-deficiency syndrome. The concept that there could actually be hundreds of variations contributing to more subtle, but nevertheless clinically relevant, examples of abnormal immune-system function was not really appreciated or talked about. Now that so much has been worked out about the function of the immune system generally and as we begin to understand the role of genetic SNP/mutation variability of the many, many proteins and the effect of external environmental toxins on the immune system, we are beginning to understand the much more complex ways that immune-system dysfunction occurs. This is also allowing new and effective treatments to restore and maintain more normal immune-system function, which allows better ways of dealing with infection threats.

The Important and Underappreciated Role of Stealth Infections in Chronic Inflammation

We are learning more and more each day about the concept of stealth infections. Stealth infection is a term applied to a situation whereby an infectious agent, whether it be a virus, a bacteria, a fungus, or a parasite, is able to remain in some form in the body after initial infection. Think of the recent ads on television proclaiming that "if you have had the chicken pox, the virus is still inside you." Other examples include the herpes-simplex virus, which is capable of causing recurrent oral herpes sores, or the bacteria *borrelia burgdorferi* capable of causing ongoing and chronic Lyme disease. There is also the Epstein-Barr viral infection with certain type of lymphoma and the measles virus with delayed-onset measles, which can cause encephalitis. This list continues to grow. As you can see from the list above, the possibilities of infectious-disease agents lingering inside our bodies, possibly for months if not years and decades, is something to be considered as a potential cause for ongoing, chronic-inflammation-associated diseases. In fact, there are those who would argue that most of the agents that infect us may actually remain in a stealth infection role. I think it is fair to say that we all have foreign infectious attackers in our bodies at all times. I don't believe that this is anything new, although I think that there is a real possibility that this is becoming a bigger problem as time progresses. The infectious agents have acquired unique and novel mechanisms to remain in their stealth roles including use of biofilms, spores, encapsulation, and intracellular existence where they avoid detection by elements of the immune system; they will even insert their genetic materials (DNA and RNA) into our own only to reemerge at some future time.

The prospect of killing these critters in their stealth guises with synthetic drugs is daunting, if not outright impossible. There is no question that antibiotics can sometimes play a very useful role in at least suppressing the numbers of and activities of some of these infectious agents in some circumstances. There may be circumstances where natural, plant-derived substances with known anti-infective powers may also play safe and useful roles in suppressing and controlling infection, including stealth infections. The critical role of an optimally functioning immune system, armed with its full array of capabilities and unencumbered by loss of capacity due to environmental toxins, nutrient deficiencies, hormonal imbalance, sleep loss, and undernourishment continues to be of vital importance.

One area of my personal interest that received almost no attention in my traditional medical training but now we know is a very important and yet currently incompletely understood is known as immune disruption by infectious agents. This principle actually makes perfect sense when you think about. The underlying principle here is that some germs that attack us have actually learned—whether or not a virus or bacteria can learn is a semantic argument anyway—or at least acquired the ability to take steps to disrupt, distract, depress, or otherwise disenable the immune system. One interesting example of this is the enzyme nagalase (alpha-N-acetylgalactosaminidase) which is a protein enzyme made by certain viruses and cancer cells that catalyzes an enzymatic reaction that breaks down and inactivates an important human protein known as Gc protein-derived macrophage activating factor or Gc-MAF. Gc-MAF is a necessary protein for normal immune activity. It is made by cleaving off a portion of the vitamin D receptor protein. The role of nagalase and Gc-MAF in immune-system disruption is only one example of cases where infectious agents can impair the immune-system activity designed to deal with them.

In conclusion, the injury that we sustain from the various causes of inflammation and infection, which together cause chronic symptoms, chronic diseases, and premature aging of our tissues, is a truly fascinating and complex situation that must be understood and addressed in our quest to achieve true health and wellness. Degradation of our modern-day environment is causing this endeavor to be progressively more difficult. I have years of experience and have studied these various mechanisms and treatment modalities, both traditional and nontraditional, and I have applied them in thousands of individual cases. For those who are continuing to experience illness and have not been able to receive adequate care, I urge you to find a health-care provider who is versed in the principles that I have outlined in this chapter.

CHAPTER 8

Nourishment: You Are What You Eat

During my education in Western medicine when I attended one of the premier medical schools in the country, I received a very minimal amount of learning about diet, nutrition, and associated pathological conditions. We studied about the traditional vitamin-deficiency diseases like scurvy, beriberi, rickets, megaloblastic anemia, Korsakoff's syndrome, kwashiorkor, and other esoteric conditions that I have never really seen in my thirty-plus years of practice. We didn't discuss the vast amount of disease associated with more minor, but nevertheless troubling, deficiencies, imbalances, and metabolic-pathway abnormalities that I now see in my practice almost every day. In those days, there was almost nothing known about the role that genetics and epigenetics played in disorders of diet and nutrition. We spent essentially no time talking about the growing amount of external environmental toxins that interfere with our nutrition and metabolism. We never discussed the role of the human microbiome, the vast number of species and individual organisms that live in our intestine and play a huge role in our nutritional status. Honestly, I believe that at the time, much of the science did not exist, and the science that did exist was deemed to be of minimal importance by our mentors. Since then, I have learned enough about diet and nutrition to fill several textbooks on the subject, and new information is coming at a truly astounding rate of speed by the day.

Nutrients Lack of Respect in Western Medicine

From my present perspective, I now understand that by paying attention to the large number of ways that our biological systems can fail to function in an ideal way, it is possible to intervene in ways that can start to restore ideal function. The complexity of this endeavor cannot be overstated. To really succeed, one literally needs to have a fundamental understanding of the total of human metabolism. I have a poster on the wall of my consultation room that measures twenty-by-thirty inches and is filled in very small print with only a portion of our metabolic pathways. I sometimes jokingly tell my patients that there will be an exam at the end of the consult. I really mostly display the poster just to present the enormity and complexity of the issue. Research, including the recently completed human-genome project, suggests that humans possess over one thousand unique protein enzymes responsible for facilitating over twenty-five hundred different metabolic reactions.

It is somewhat difficult to try to summarize the principles of nutritional therapy in a handbook or introduction like this. Brevity requires that I only hit the high points.

The Cure Is in the Kitchen: The Role of Diet in Chronic Disease

I almost always start the care of a new patient suffering from chronic disease with a discussion about diet. There is a name for our modern Western diet. We refer to it as SAD—standard American diet. Although it's meant to be a bit facetious, it is actually quite appropriate. Our modern diet is a consequence of our hurry-up, multitasking lifestyle as presented by the profit-motivated food-producing conglomerate businesses that have managed to insert themselves into our daily routines. The negative effects on our biological systems are enormous. Think of the daily consumption of diet cola and packaged foods with long lists of ingredients like monosodium glutamate, high-fructose corn syrup, and a variety of artificial flavors, colors, texturizers, and preservatives, which are usually written in text too small to read with the naked eye. I know you get the picture.

I start by telling patients that in order to be truly well, they have to stop taking in the toxins that are literally killing them. The first principle is to start eating chemical-free, real food. I tell them that I want them to eat food that their great, great grandmother would recognize as food and not packaged, freeze-dried, or thoroughly processed foods. I advise them to eat as organically as they can afford, realizing that, unfortunately, today there is a real price premium on food that is produced with our health in mind.

The mainstream dietary recommendations from the seventies, including the food pyramid, came mostly from groups like the Dairyman's Association, the Beef Council, and other organizations with their own agendas that did not always include our health and wellness high on the list. I have been amazed, but not surprised, to see the gradual morphing of dietary recommendations by various health organizations and the government, especially in recent years. The Dietary Guidelines Advisory Committee just recently released a draft of their 2015 guidelines that states, in essence, that dietary cholesterol was not so bad after all. Who would have thought?

I tell my patients to eat mostly plants. Green, leafy vegetables are nutrient rich, especially when they have not been recently sprayed with pesticides and other harmful chemicals. It's good to eat all the colors of the rainbow when it comes to vegetables and fruits. Many of the natural substances that impart color to fruits and vegetables are valuable phytonutrients that play important roles in our biological processes. I encourage limitation of carbohydrates. Most people think of sugar when I say carbs, and I must usually point out that there is actually a much higher density of sugar, glucose, in many starches than in table sugar. I tell folks that the right kind of fats are not only OK to eat, but that many of the right fats are actually required for good health and normal metabolism. Think of the beneficial effect of omega-3 and omega-7 fatty acids—as in marine oil—macadamia nuts, and the medium-chain triglycerides in things like coconut oil, which provide a simple energy source for our millions of mitochondria that we use to power virtually all of our metabolic activities.

The history of the development of diet recommendations for chronic, inflammation-induced disease, including food allergy, is very colorful to say the least. Many of the early introducers were quickly dismissed as being unscientific, and their diets were often summarily dismissed. It's worth looking at some of the individual case histories to understand the power that organized forces can quickly generate in order to maintain the status quo.

A Brief Historical Look at Healing Diets

There are a number of different diets that have become popular over the years that help people suffering from chronic, inflammation-induced illnesses. Dr. Ben Feingold, an allergist from San Francisco, California, published a book in 1974 titled *Why Your Child Is Hyperactive*. This book became the origin of the Feingold Diet. Dr. Feingold advocated that a number of food additives and chemicals, including aspirin and salicylates in food, contributed to hyperactivity in children based on his extensive observations. Although his diet still has many adherents today and I commonly recommend avoidance of food additive chemicals, he was ridiculed by many authorities in his day.

In the late seventies and early eighties, Dr. William Crook expanded on the work of Dr. Orian Truss and popularized the yeast-free diet in his 1983 book, *The Yeast Connection*. He found that many patients with chronic illness seemed to benefit significantly from a low-sugar diet and antiyeast medicines like nystatin. It was his hypothesis that the common intestinal yeast, *candida albicans*, was playing a causal role. Dr. Crook's yeast-free diet or variations of it continue to be recommended for patients by many integrative, functional, and holistic providers.

I tend to routinely recommend the Paleo Diet, which is based on the hypothetical diet of early Paleolithic-period, human hunter-gatherers. This period, also known as the Stone Age, spanned from about 2.6 million years ago until about 10,000 years ago. It ended before humans began to live in stationary communities, before they practiced farming of the grass grains like corn and wheat, and before the domestication of grazing animals. This diet basically consists of vegetables and tubers, fruits, small game, fish, and nuts. Stone Age man also ate insects. I don't get too many takers on that part of the diet. It does not allow refined sugars and most starches, especially the cereal grains. The Paleo Diet comes in many forms and variations that are largely similar, and each one has its own group of advocates.

I also spend time talking to people about eating slowly and chewing thoroughly. I think it is important to enjoy eating. Too often, meal time is seen as time wasted because we race through our daily routines. One of the advantages of drinking blended smoothies, I believe, relies on the fact the blending process significantly enhances more complete digestion just as thorough chewing does. It is also important to limit portion size, and this is much easier to do when we eat slowly and allow time for the natural signals of satiety to be generated. Often, eating a number of small meals is helpful in this regard.

Food Allergies and Intolerances in Chronic, Inflammation-Based Disease

Since food allergies and intolerances play a major role in contributing to chronic, inflammation-based disease, I spend a significant amount of time working with patients on this area of their pathologies. I had a keen interest in allergy even before I began to transition away from traditional medicine toward a more functional and holistic direction as an otolaryngic allergist. I can sum up food-allergy treatment in two words—it's complicated. I don't say this to be cute. It really is complicated and very controversial as well. There is controversy about the definitions, the testing, the pathophysiology, the treatments, the diets, and the results of treatment interventions. I know you get the picture.

I can just say that, because of the complexity of the issue, it is important to individualize the approach to each patient based on many different factors. I take special care with individuals with a history that suggests a possible tendency toward food-induced anaphylaxis. This is the type of food allergy associated with histamine release, swelling, hives, itching, and shortness of breath that can become life-threatening. This type of food allergy is best managed by someone who is well versed in this type of allergy and its management. I definitely don't treat all food allergies the same way even though the principles of treatment that I use are, for me, well established.

The Role of the Microbiome (Our Intestinal Bugs) in Health and Disease

Consider this: when we eat a meal or snack, we are not only feeding ourselves, but we are also feeding the diverse group of hitchhikers who reside in our intestinal tracts, or intestinal microbiome. Some new research is indicating that dietary changes cause rather rapid and dramatic shifts in the numbers and species of germs and other microbes in our gut. The makeup of this potpourri of microorganisms has significant ramifications for our digestive function, our intestinal health, and our health and wellness in general. We are also learning that our cravings for certain foods, for example sweets, and beverages, say alcohol, are directly caused by signaling molecules that are made by germs in the gut that trigger signals to the brain that make us want to eat or drink certain things. So, in a sense, we are at least in part controlled by our intestinal microbiomes.

One of the most important reasons that I spend a significant amount of time and energy on my patients' digestive and intestinal health stems from my awareness that the gut is the source of most inflammation that affects the body systemically. When you think about the nature of the gut, it makes perfect sense. The gut is a hollow tube that travels from our mouths to our anuses. If you were to spread it out all the way, it would have a surface area about the size of a tennis court due to the many convolutions. Everything inside the lumen of our gut is really outside our bodies. Within the intestine, the barrier between the external environment and the inside of our bodies is actually the complex intestinal lining. The external environment within the lumen, the hollow part of the intestine, is quite inhospitable. It is a dark, low-oxygen, moist, warm environment filled with energy-rich molecules and trillions of germs from hundreds of different species. This lining has to be a semi-permeable barrier, which means that it must allow certain nutrients to come in and yet act as a barrier to prevent the entrance of harmful substances. As compared to the gut lining, the skin has a really easy job. It's really just a barrier to keep out foreign stuff, provide some structural framework, and not allow anything important to leak out.

Understanding Leaky Gut

To assist the gut in coping with this difficult task, about 70 percent of the cells of our immune system are arrayed just inside the gut lining and within a few millimeters of the gut lumen. Much of the disease that my patients suffer from is a direct consequence of a loss of the normal barrier function of the gut. The term leaky gut was talked about for years only to be dismissed by many traditional medical scientists and doctors. Today, thanks to sophisticated study and experimentation, the concept of altered intestinal permeability, or leaky gut, is widely accepted, and its role in inflammation-induced disease is considered foundational to our understanding of many diseases. I explain to my patients that leaky gut arises as a consequence of three main factors: first, damage caused by the effects of chemical toxins in food and water; second, the consumption of food and water that we are allergic, or otherwise intolerant to, from an immune perspective; and third, intestinal dysbiosis, which is a term given to the disorder that results from the presence of microbes within the intestinal lumen that cause injury to the lining by virtue of their activities, metabolisms, and the substances that they excrete. In order to have a healthy gut with digestion that is conducive to ideal health, we must deal with all three of these separate factors.

The process of restoration to normal gut-barrier permeability, normalization of intestinal immune-system activation that results from this abnormal gut leakiness, and the normalization of the digestive process and nutrient absorption is a complex endeavor that must be individualized based on each patient's circumstances. History and physical exams, often augmented with functional tests of stool or blood, play key roles in determining appropriate treatments in each case. Diet modification, probiotics, prebiotics, treatment of food sensitivities, elimination of toxins, and in some cases, anti-infective agents—both natural and prescription—are the tools necessary to be successful in restoring normal intestinal health and function.

Supplementing with Vitamins and Nutrients

What about vitamin and nutrient supplementation? The science of nutrition is the subject of textbooks on its own. I am going to cover some of the fundamental ideas without making any attempt to present a treatise on vitamins and macronutrients; that would not serve my purpose. There are many great nutritional references out there. I am going to try to discuss some of the areas where nutritional issues come up almost every day in my clinical practice.

I am frequently asked by folks whether they can get all the nutrients they need simply by eating the right diet. I can certainly understand the benefit of doing this if it were possible. Unfortunately, in most cases, I don't believe that it is possible. I do believe that in most every case, the natural nutrients are in most usable forms and most highly bioavailable when they are absorbed by our digestive system when we eat real food. The problem has to do with the gradual nutrient-depleting evolution of our foods—even real food coupled with the changing nutrient needs of our bodies in the twenty-first century due to progressive environmental degradation.

If anyone can maintain a high state of sustained wellness with diet alone as the source of their nutrition, it would be an individual who has a fortuitous genome background, a low-stress lifestyle, healthy sleep patterns, regular physical exercise, a relatively low body-fat percentage, low ongoing environmental-toxin exposure, and has already been eating a very healthy diet in the past. It would have to be someone who currently enjoys very good health with no symptoms or signs of chronic inflammation. If this sounds like you, awesome! This individual would, of course, have to continue that very healthy eating plan. This does not sound like 99 percent of the folks I see in my office every day. It is fairly common for my patients, as they become well, to see that with a healthy diet and lifestyle, their vitamin supplementation requirements go way down. I work with individuals who have progressed with our assistance to experience true health, and at that point, the program becomes one of sustaining that wellness and optimizing (delaying) aging-related decline.

I do have a strong opinion about the amount of supplementation and the quality of supplementation that an individual typically requires. Most of the folks who come to my office for the first time have been suffering for a while and have typically been seen by a number of other health-care providers from various disciplines and backgrounds before seeing me. It is very common for a patient to come into my office for the first visit carrying a large bag filled with a significant number of various vitamin, mineral, and herbal preparations from a variety of makers. I know that the monthly expense associated with this personal pharmacy is often substantial. Many of these patients also have a good number of bottles of prescription medicines as well. I always tell folks that I am not helping them very much if they get well but go broke in the process. I try to be very cost conscious in everything I do to help the individuals that I treat. It is always my goal to consolidate, eliminate, and reduce supplements and synthetic medications, as much as safely possible, to still reach the patient's desired goals. I have this same philosophy of value when it comes to recommending diagnostic testing as well.

I want to be careful not to step on toes here. I have seen instances where it might have appeared that recommendations of others may have been related to an agenda greater than the patient's real wellness. That's all I will say about that. You can read it as you will.

So what can I say about nutrients and natural, plant-based medicines in general? I need to say that supplement needs must be individualized. Today, with the knowledge of gene SNP/mutation-caused abnormalities of enzymes, we are able to predict with greater accuracy than ever before which supplements will be most beneficial and which supplements might be intolerable to a particular individual. We now know that vitamins and certain nutrients can only perform their necessary functions if they exist in a certain form or state. Probably the best known example is with the nutrient folic acid/folate/vitamin B9. We also know that most vitamin and cofactor activity occurs inside our cells, and therefore, considerable thought needs to be applied to how to get the necessary factors *inside the specific cells where they are needed*. For instance, you are not going to help someone suffering from neuron dysfunction related to folate deficiency until you are able to deliver the appropriate, active form of folate into the body, across the blood-brain barrier, and across the neuron cell membrane and into the cell with the need.

Assessing Vitamins and Nutrients

This also brings up an important point about measuring vitamin levels. The circulating amount of an inactive or even counteractive form of a vitamin or cofactor in the urine, blood, or serum may tell you almost nothing about the action of the active form(s) of that vitamin within the cells that are not functioning optimally. You really have to understand what you are testing, or you can reach unhelpful conclusions that result in unhelpful recommendations for treatment.

When an essential nutrient playing a vital role in a given metabolic pathway is deficient, the body uses a sophisticated form of coping known as homeostasis.

Homeostasis is the way that the body tries to make the most of a bad situation. It makes adjustments to reduce the abnormal function of the pathway. If the nutrient in question is returned to the system and the pathway is opened up when it was not previously, it is common to see a rapid change in the homeostasis of the cell. This can sometimes result in dramatic changes that may cause rapid swings in symptoms and functions. In order to accommodate this, I have learned that it is best to introduce different medications, vitamins, minerals, phytonutrients, and others *one at a time and gradually*. If the introduction of an agent causes troubling changes, it is possible that it will not be tolerated in that form by the body, but it is much more likely that it will ultimately be tolerated, and in fact beneficial, once the homeostasis setting has reset. This phenomenon is sometimes referred to as regressive healing.

What about vitamin testing? Nutrient assessment in the body is the subject of volumes of numerous good textbooks, and it isn't my goal to cover testing to that depth; however, some general observations are in order. There are many ways to assess nutrient activity in the body. Certainly the amount of a nutrient can be measured in a variety of ways. One must consider, as in the discussion above, that a vitamin or other nutrient might exist in a number of states or forms, and this must be taken into account. For example, the levels in the blood of 25-hydroxy vitamin D and 1,25-hydroxy vitamin D are not interchangeable and must be interpreted differently. Whether the nutrient is being measured in hair, saliva, urine, stool, sweat, serum, whole blood, capillary blood, or RBCs, red blood cells, may give very different results. The actual nutrient levels may not correlate with the functional activity of the nutrient typically inside the cell or even inside the subcellular organelle, the mitochondrion, for example. Sometimes the total body stores of a nutrient might be desirable to know. Urine testing can involve random testing, first-morning void, twenty-four-hour collection, and in the case of toxic minerals, chelating, agent-provoked sampling might yield more useful information.

In some cases, trying to measure the level of a particular nutrient is either impossible, expensive, difficult, or unreliable. In these situations, it may be desirable to assess the nutrient functional activity in another way. There are many ways that this is done. In some cases, measurement of various metabolic markers—metabolic end-products, intermediates, or excretory products—from various metabolic pathways can give useful information about nutrient activity. For example, measuring the serum level of methylmalonic acid is a good way to assess vitamin-B12 activity. There are also various, elegant cell-functional assays on the market that use different models to evaluate nutrient functional activity at the cellular level.

The bottom line is that there is not just one way to assess a vitamin, cofactor, or other nutrient, and one must also consider the manner and circumstances under which the assessment is done. There are certainly situations where one way to approach a specific vitamin or supplement is by a trial. In other words, if the clinical picture of an individual suggests a significant probability of deficiency of a given nutrient and supplementing that nutrient is known to be safe, then a perfectly acceptable approach would be to supplement the individual with the nutrient in question and carefully observe the clinical outcome. This same approach is, in fact, also performed daily and has been for years by traditional physicians using traditional synthetic prescriptions in a number of different clinical circumstances for a host of different symptoms and diseases. It may not seem that scientific, but it often works, and it's generally safe.

CHAPTER 9

Exercise: Use It or Lose It!

The *e* in *got to shine* stands for exercise, and I include any movement and stretching activity in that. This includes aerobic as well as resistance-training exercise. I always add the caveat that one can only exercise as he or she is able.

There is an abundance of evidence that convincingly shows that vigorous physical activity, done properly and not excessively, clearly contributes to disease recovery and sustained wellness in most situations, including virtually all chronic, inflammation-induced diseases. The corollary that absence of regular vigorous physical activity contributes to many diseases is also true.

Maintaining a consistent program of physical training is as important to achieving true health and sustaining wellness as eating a healthy diet, taking the proper supplemental vitamins and nutrients, maintaining appropriate levels of critical hormones essential for maintaining normal cellular function, and maintaining a program to reduce and relieve mental stress. It has also been clearly proven that exercising the mind is also essential to maintaining health, cognitive function, and balance into later life. The rather dramatic improvement in athletic performance and world sports performance records has come as a result of better programs of training and nutrition. This accomplishment in the background of progressive environmental degradation is really remarkable and points out the benefits of ongoing programs of training and nutrition.

Let's explore just some of the science that shows how beneficial consistent physical training is to our health, longevity, and performance. In a large global study published in the Lancet medical journal researchers found that inactivity accounted for 5.3 million of 57 million global deaths in 2008. The researchers commented that a 10% to 25% reduction in global rates of inactivity would result in global reduction of 500,000 to 1.3 million deaths from all causes annually. Physical activity protects telormeres, the small protective caps on chromosomes that have been corelated with aging and death according to a study from the University of California at San Francisco. A study from the University of Otago in New Zealand found that when middle aged and older adults were separated into five groups based on fitness assessment, 25% of the individuals in the least fit group died compared to 6% of individuals in the most fit group over a nine year period.

Frailty is a medical condition associated with vulnerability due to an increased risk of injury from falls, hospitalization, cognitive decline, and psychological stress. A study from the Institut Universitaire de Geriatrie de Montreal concluded that physical exercise training improved cognitive function and psychological well-being in frail older adults.

A study from the University of Pittsburgh by Mertz and colleagues published in 2010 demonstrated that regular exercise reduced the risk of falls with two hours of aerobic exercise per week exerting the greatest protective effect. Men with low fitness levels were over twice as likely to fall compared to men in the high fitness level group.

Researchers from the University of Western Sydney in Australia studied a group of 91,375 Australians over age 65 and concluded that there is a significant positive relationship between physical activity and physical function in older adults. They demonstrated that older adults who were more physically active were less likely to experience functional limitation compared to more sedentary seniors.

A study published in 2012 by Toker and colleagues from the University of Tel Aviv in Israel found that individuals who participate in regular physical activity are less likely to experience depression and work-related burnout as compared to less physically active individuals. A similar study performed at Penn State University found that folks who were more physically active reported greater levels of excitement and enthusiasm than those who were less active. A number of studies have clearly demonstrated the role of regular physical exercise with brain and cognitive health. Even in childhood exercise has been shown to be important in getting a headstart on learning and cognitive development. Physical inactivity has been demonstrated as a contributing factor to poorer academic performance and performance on neuropsychological tests. At the same time participation in regular exercise programs demonstrates improved memory, attention, and decision-making. Science has shown that regular exercise promotes the growth of new nerve cells and improves the microcirculation to the brain. It also appears to enhance the production of important beneficial brain chemicals such as brain derived neurotrophic factor (BDNF) and insulin growth factor-1 (IGF-1) which have been shown to promote brain cell growth, differentiation, and repair. Researchers from China Medical University Hospital in Taiwan discovered that exercise promotes neurogenesis which has a positive effect on mood and cognition especially in the brain's hippocampus, an area involved in memory and emotional regulation.

In 2011 the World Health Organization identified that physical inactivity is the fourth leading risk factor for global mortality and that global inactivity is rising in many countries worldwide. In this report the WHO issued recommendations that individuals aged 18-64 should perform at least 150 minutes of moderate-intensity aerobic exercise or at least 75 minutes of vigorous-intensity aerobic exercise throughout the week. They went on to recommend that individuals should engage in muscle-strengthening activities involving major muscle groups two or more days per week.

In regards to strength training it is now known that folks typically lose about 30% of their muscle strength between the ages of 50 and 70 years and that it is critical to maintain health and mobility to preserve muscle strength as we age. Researchers at the University of Potsdam in Germany found that regular strength or resistance training at least three or four times per week increased muscle strength and reduced muscle atrophy. Their research showed that in order to increase muscle mass, repetitions that were 60-85% of the one-repetition max were needed and that higher intensities were needed to increase rapidly available muscle stremgth and retain motor function. German research also finds that regular physical exercise activates the important enzyme telomerase which stabilizes the chromosome telomeres and extends longevity.

Important tenants of training stress full range of motion encouraging balance and symmetry. Attention should be paid to upper and lower extremities as well as the neck, shoulders, back, chest, and core. The use of the exercise ball is a good way to work the core and works to strengthen and tone the many small muscle groups in the hips, back, and abdomen.

Thanks to my twenty years in the US Army medical corps, I have been obligated to maintain an active and regular routine of physical training so I can personally attest to its benefits. I don't really consider the instruction of patients on the specifics of implementation of physical training to be an area of expertise for me. This is one of the areas where I depend heavily on the expertise of others. Fortunately, there are many good physical trainers, physical therapists, kinesiologists, and other coaches and guides in almost every community.

I am not advocating training for a triathlon. In fact, I believe training can be overdone and can contribute to tissue injury, illnesses, and symptoms. I also believe that, like many things, physical training needs to be gradually introduced after other aspects of healing have been addressed first. It is not wise, and it will be harmful and unsuccessful to introduce this too early and too quickly.

Fitness training is very stress relieving when it is done right. When comingled with a program of deep breathing, relaxation, and meditation, it is especially able to eliminate disease-causing stress.

I believe that a combination of resistance training, like lifting weights, and aerobic training is best. The exact number of days of the week and minutes per day is controversial, and I like to leave that up to the patient and the trainer. There are a wide variety of different types of resistance training just as there are many types of aerobic training. There is training that can be performed inside and outside and even on the go.

Balance, stability, strength, and endurance are important in almost all sports activities. Maintaining high levels of physical activity extends life and reduces the incidence of many chronic inflammation-based diseases. The researchers at the University of Texas-Southwestern Medical Center (my alma mater) determined that the fittest study participants had dramatically lower healthcare costs by 36-40% compared to the least-fit group.

The key is to commit to a regular program that can become a part of your daily activities. The patients that I see doing this regularly report on the perceived benefits, and that has certainly been true for me.

CHAPTER 10

Conclusion: You Can Do This!

I sincerely hope that this handbook has not caused anyone to be intimidated or discouraged from committing to embarking on the journey to true health and sustained wellness. The integrative, functional, alternative, and holistic model does present a long process that must be carried out slowly and methodically to be successful. I tell my patients that they are running a marathon race, not a fifty-yard dash. The Western medicine episodic-care model of one symptom and one prescription has no place here. I sometimes use the analogy of peeling an onion one layer at a time. I find that when I have my patients tackle too many issues at once, they often feel much worse by getting frustrated and, sometimes, confused. It is preferable to proceed slowly and methodically.

I believe it is important to start by a concerted effort to stop the onslaught of toxic stresses entering the body. By avoiding sources of toxic chemicals in the air, food, and water we can at least reduce the rate of injury caused by these sources. I am sure that there is much we should be doing collectively as a community to reduce our exposures generally. I have been gratified to see the many grassroots organizations that are springing up with agendas to clean up the various sources of toxic stress in our environment. There remains much to be done if we are going to reverse the progressive amount of exposure that up until now is increasing rapidly. If not for us then let's at least do it for our future generations!

Once we stop the intake of various toxins and stresses, we can then begin to slowly and carefully remove the various internal substances and factors that contribute to disease. At the same time we can determine and replace those necessary nutrients, vitamins, minerals, and cofactors that our bodies need to function optimally.

Now, thanks to completion of the human genome project, personalized and affordable genome analysis is ready for prime time. With President Obama's call for funding for his precision medicine initiative early in 2015 this exciting area of discovery will progress rapidly. I currently use a saliva-based test to analyze a number of critical genes controlling a number of vital human metabolic enzymes. The information that I get from this testing has proven very useful in assisting individuals in finding detours around some of their genetically inherited metabolic road-blocks.

I don't pretend to have all the answers for everyone. I don't believe anyone does. I do, however, have many more answers than I did coming out of medical school. I have many more answers than I did when I began to study the principles of integrative medicine. I have many more answers than I did ten years ago—or even five years ago. I know, too, that I will have many more answers as time progresses. I also know that I have a strong commitment and passion to assist my patients and others to achieve true health, joy, productivity, and sustained wellness. I am committed to never giving up on anyone and pursuing answers when no answers are readily found.

If in reading this guidebook you feel a certain motivation to take the journey to reach the true health and sustained wellness that is there for you, consider this my challenge for you. Engage the services of a healer or group of healers who can assist you in the journey.

I also believe that there is a loving creator, God, of the universe who loves us and wants only good for us. I depend on the Spirit's help every day in my work as a healer. I firmly believe that with God's help, all things are possible and that the decision to start the journey to health and wellness is the most important commitment that anyone can make. Your most important investment is *you!*

About the Author

After finishing his formal education at the University of Texas at Austin and Southwestern medical school in Dallas, Dr. Taylor entered military service in the US Army and served as an ear, nose, and throat surgeon. He then settled with his family in Alamosa, Colorado, where he provided ENT care for twenty years. While treating patients in Colorado, he began to routinely interact with people suffering from severe chronic diseases like autism and autoimmunity and severe allergic and inflammatory conditions. He found that all the standard treatments that he and his medical colleagues had been taught in school did not significantly benefit these chronically ill patients. Driven by frustration and a confidence that there were answers, he began a process of further health education that focused on environmental medicine and antiaging medicine.

Gradually, over twenty-five years, his practice style has evolved into an integrative/functional one that focuses on a combination of the best of Western medicine integrated with modern care whose aim is to utilize the body's natural systems of detoxification and repair to restore health and maintain true wellness. Dr. Taylor has learned that traditional organized medicine's approach of sickness medicine, where every symptom requires a different prescription and side effects require even more prescriptions, is not adequate for the chronic diseases so many of us face today.

Dr. Taylor says, "I get much satisfaction when my care assists kids who are nonverbal to talk, women who are fatigued and in pain to feel truly well, and older patients who are experiencing declining mental function to enjoy life again."

Dr. Taylor lives in Austin, Texas, where he enjoys spending time with his wife, grown children, and two beautiful granddaughters. He enjoys photography, cycling, and travel when he isn't taking care of patients.

Dr. Taylor is currently accepting new patients in his Austin, Texas clinic. Appointments can be scheduled by calling 512-800-5309.

Visit Dr Taylor's website: www.TexasIntegrative.com for more information about his services.

www.ingramcontent.com/pod-product-compliance
Lightning Source LLC
Chambersburg PA
CBHW070608290526
45790CB00002B/830